MYOMECTOMY
BEFORE AND AFTER

By

Michelle F. Spencer

Copyright © 2023 Michelle F. Spencer

All rights reserved. No part of this book may be reproduced, stored in a retrieval system, or transmitted in any form or by any means, electronic, mechanical, photocopying, recording, scanning, or otherwise, without the prior written permission of the publisher.

This book is a work of non-fiction. The views expressed herein are the sole responsibility of the author and do not necessarily reflect the views of the publisher or its agents.

Table of Contents:

Table of Contents:

Chapter 1

Introduction to Myomectomy
    What is a Myomectomy?
    Benefits of Myomectomy

Chapter 2

Types of Myomectomy
    Abdominal Myomectomy
    Laparoscopic Myomectomy
    Hysteroscopic Myomectomy

Chapter 3

Pre-Operative Care
    Before Surgery
    During Surgery
    After Surgery

Chapter 4

Risks and Complications

Chapter 5

RECOVERY
    Physical Recovery
    Emotional Recovery

Chapter 6

Recovery and Follow-up
- Hospital Stay
- Follow-up Appointments
- Diet
- Activity

Chapter 7

Conclusion

Chapter 1

Introduction to Myomectomy

There was a woman named Jane who had been struggling with infertility for years. No matter what she tried, she could not get pregnant. After consulting with her doctor, she learned that she had a condition called fibroids, or non-cancerous tumors in her uterus. Her doctor suggested that she undergo a procedure called a myomectomy to remove the fibroids.

Jane was scared and uncertain about the procedure, but she knew that it was her only hope for having a child. She gathered her courage and prepared for the surgery.

On the day of the surgery, Jane was surrounded by doctors and nurses who were there to make sure she was safe. She was given anaesthesia, and once she was asleep, the doctors began the myomectomy. They carefully removed the fibroids from her uterus, taking great care not to damage any of the surrounding tissue.

When the surgery was complete, Jane felt relieved. She had been so worried that something could go wrong, but the doctors had done a great job and she was feeling better already. After a few weeks of recovery, Jane was able to go home and start trying to have a baby.

Months later, Jane was finally able to announce that she was pregnant. She was overjoyed at the news and immediately thanked her doctor for performing the myomectomy. She knew that without it, she would never have been able to conceive.

Jane's story is an example of how a myomectomy can help some women who are struggling to get pregnant. Although it is a serious procedure and should not be taken lightly, it can have a positive impact on a woman's life. Jane's story is proof of that.

What is a Myomectomy?

Uterine fibroids, which are benign tumors of the uterus, can be surgically removed by surgery known as a myomectomy. Myomectomy can be done using several different techniques, including open surgery, laparoscopy, hysteroscopy, and robotic surgery. The type of surgery chosen will depend on the size and location of the fibroids, as well as the patient's overall health and fertility goals.

The goal of myomectomy is to remove the fibroids while leaving the uterus intact. This can help preserve fertility and reduce the risk of complications during pregnancy. Myomectomy may also reduce heavy menstrual bleeding and other symptoms associated with fibroids.

Recovery from myomectomy can vary depending on the type of procedure and the patient's overall health. Generally, patients are advised to rest for several weeks and are encouraged to take pain medications as prescribed by their doctor. After the procedure, regular follow-up appointments with a gynaecologist are recommended to monitor any remaining fibroids and the patient's overall health.

Myomectomy is a safe and effective treatment for uterine fibroids. However, the fibroids may grow back after the procedure, and the patient may need to consider other treatments if the fibroids persist or recur.

Benefits of Myomectomy

The surgical removal of uterine fibroids is known as a myomectomy. It is usually recommended for women who have large fibroids or who have symptoms that cannot be managed with medication.

The benefits of having a myomectomy include:

1. Relief from painful symptoms caused by fibroids, such as heavy bleeding, pelvic pain, and pressure in the abdomen.

2. Improved fertility. Fibroids can interfere with the implantation of an embryo or make it difficult for a woman to become pregnant. A myomectomy can remove fibroids that are blocking the fallopian tubes or prevent a fertilized egg from implanting in the uterus.

3. Reduced risk of miscarriage. Fibroids can increase a woman's risk of having a miscarriage. Removing them can help reduce this risk.

4. Reduced risk of preterm labour. Fibroids can increase a woman's risk of going into labour prematurely. A myomectomy can reduce this risk.

5. Reduced risk of Cesarean section. Fibroids can make it difficult for a baby to pass through the birth canal. Removing them can reduce the risk of needing a C-section.

Chapter 2

Types of Myomectomy

Abdominal Myomectomy

Abdominal myomectomy is a surgical procedure that removes uterine fibroids, which are noncancerous growths located in the muscular wall of the uterus. The procedure is performed through an abdominal incision and involves cutting the fibroids away from the uterus and removing them from the body.

During the procedure, the uterus itself is usually left intact, although some of the surrounding tissue may be removed to ensure that all of the fibroids are removed. The recovery time for abdominal myomectomy varies, depending on the size and number of fibroids removed, as well as the patient's overall health. Typically, patients can expect to return to normal activities within four to six weeks.

Laparoscopic Myomectomy

Uterine fibroids can be removed by a less invasive surgical technique called a laparoscopic myomectomy. It is often done using laparoscopic tools, which are inserted through small incisions in the abdomen.

The doctor uses a camera to view the organs, and a special instrument to cut and remove the fibroids. The surgeon may also use sutures to close the uterus and prevent bleeding. Under general anaesthesia, this procedure normally takes two hours. The recovery time is usually shorter than with an open myomectomy.

Hysteroscopic Myomectomy

Uterine fibroids are removed using a surgery called a hysteroscopic myomectomy. It is a minimally invasive procedure that is performed using a hysteroscope, which is a thin, lighted viewing instrument that is inserted into the uterus through the cervix.

During the procedure, the fibroids are removed using special instruments such as forceps, resectoscopes, and morcellators. The doctor may also use a laser to remove the fibroids. After the procedure, the patient may need to take medication to help with pain and reduce the risk of infection. Recovery time is shorter than with traditional surgery, and most patients can return to work and their normal activities within a few days.

Chapter 3

Pre-Operative Care

Pre-operative care is an essential part of the surgical process, and patients need to receive the best possible care before their surgery. Pre-operative care includes a complete medical history and physical examination, laboratory tests, and other diagnostic tests such as X-rays, CT scans, and MRI scans.

During this process, the doctor will assess your health status and determine if you are a suitable candidate for the surgery. Pre-operative care also includes providing the patient with education and instructions about the upcoming procedure and its associated risks.

The goal of pre-operative care is to ensure that you are in the best possible condition for the surgery and to reduce the risk of complications during or after the procedure.

Before Surgery

1. Pre-operative testing: This typically includes blood work, an EKG, and imaging tests such as an ultrasound or MRI to assess the size and location of the fibroids.

2. Discussing the procedure: Your doctor will discuss the details of the surgery with you, including the type of myomectomy to be performed and the risks associated with the procedure.

3. Pre-operative counselling: You may be asked to attend a pre-operative counselling session with a doctor or nurse to discuss your expectations and any concerns you may have before the surgery.

4. Pre-operative instructions: You may be given instructions by your doctor or nurse on preparing for the surgery, such as fasting before the procedure, avoiding certain medications and supplements, and discontinuing birth control.

5. Pre-operative medication: Your doctor may prescribe medication to reduce swelling and pain after the surgery.

6. Pre-operative diet: Your doctor may advise you to follow a low-sodium diet before the surgery to reduce the risk of complications.

During Surgery

1. Anesthesia is administered to the patient. Depending on the size and number of fibroids, general or regional anaesthesia may be used.

2. An incision is made in the abdomen. This can be done through traditional open surgery, laparoscopy, or a robotic-assisted procedure.

3. The fibroids are located and removed. If the fibroids are very large, sometimes the uterus is removed (hysterectomy).

4. The incision is closed and the area is cleaned.

5. The patient may be monitored during recovery and may be discharged the same day or the next day.

6. Follow-up care may include medications, lifestyle changes, and regular check-ups.

After Surgery

1. Make sure to follow your doctor's instructions for pre-operative care, such as fasting and taking medications as prescribed.

2. Stay well hydrated before the surgery and drink plenty of fluids during the recovery period.

3. Avoid strenuous activities or heavy lifting for at least 1-2 weeks following the surgery.

4. Get plenty of rest and avoid stressful activities.

5. Eat a balanced diet and take any medications as prescribed by your doctor.

6. Take steps to avoid constipation, including drinking plenty of fluids and eating a high-fibre diet.

7. Avoid sexual activity for at least 1-2 weeks following the procedure.

8. Wear loose-fitting clothing and avoid using tampons for at least 1-2 weeks post-surgery.

9. Follow all instructions for wound care, including gently cleaning the area, changing dressings as needed, and avoiding hot baths or swimming for at least 2 weeks.

10. Contact your doctor if you experience any unusual symptoms after the surgery, such as fever, excessive pain, or heavy bleeding.

Chapter 4

Risks and Complications

1. Bleeding: Excessive bleeding is the most common complication of myomectomy surgery. This can occur due to the cutting of the uterus and surrounding tissue.

2. Damage to the surrounding tissue: If the surgeon is not careful, the incision can damage surrounding organs, nerves, or tissue. This can result in an infection or other problems

3. Injury to the bladder or ureters: The bladder or ureters (the tubes that carry urine from the kidneys to the bladder) can be injured during the surgery. This could lead to infection and difficulty urinating.

4. Damage to the uterus: If the uterus is not closed properly after the surgery, it can lead to problems with future pregnancies.

5. Infection: Infection can occur after the surgery from germs entering the incision site. Fever, discomfort, swelling, and redness are all signs of infection.

6. Scarring: Scarring can occur after the surgery, which can make it more difficult for the uterus to expand during a future pregnancy.

7. Blood clots: Blood clots can form in the legs or lungs after the surgery, which can be a serious and life-threatening complication.

8. Anesthesia complications: Complications can occur from the use of anaesthesia during the surgery. Fever, discomfort, swelling, and redness are all signs of infection.

Chapter 5

RECOVERY

Physical Recovery

Physical recovery after a myomectomy surgery typically takes about 6-8 weeks. It is important to follow the post-operative instructions given by your doctor and give yourself plenty of time to rest and heal. The first few days after the surgery, you should limit your activity and focus on resting and taking care of yourself.

Be sure to keep the incision as clean and dry as possible. This may include taking showers instead of baths and changing dressings as needed. You should also take any medications prescribed by your doctor to help with pain and inflammation. Additionally, you should avoid any strenuous activities such as lifting, bending, and twisting for the first few weeks after your surgery.

It is important to slowly start increasing your activity level as your body begins to heal. This may include walking, light stretching, and other low-impact activities. However, be sure to listen to your body and rest when needed.

Finally, it is important to eat a healthy diet and stay hydrated. Eating a balanced diet with plenty of fruits and vegetables can help with healing and reduce inflammation. Additionally, drinking plenty of water can help keep you hydrated and reduce the risk of infection.

Overall, it is important to follow your doctor's instructions and give yourself plenty of time to rest and heal. Taking care of yourself both physically and mentally can help you recover from your myomectomy surgery and get back to your normal activities.

Emotional Recovery

Emotional recovery after myomectomy surgery is just as important as physical recovery. It can be a difficult and emotional experience for women, so it is essential to give yourself time to process your feelings. Here are some tips to help with emotional recovery:

1. Acknowledge your feelings: It is normal to feel a range of emotions after a myomectomy. Acknowledge those feelings and take the time to express them.

2. Connect with a support network: Talking to friends and family can help you to process your emotions and get support. Joining an online community or support group can also be helpful.

3. Practice self-care: Taking care of yourself can help you to manage stress and anxiety. Do things that make you feel relaxed and positive, such as exercising, meditating, or spending time in nature.

4. Seek professional help: If your emotions become overwhelming, it is important to seek help from a mental health professional. They can provide guidance and resources to help you manage your feelings.

5. Allow yourself time to heal: Give yourself time to grieve and process your emotions. Everyone's recovery is different, so don't be hard on yourself if it takes time.

Myomectomy surgery can be a challenging experience, but emotional recovery is possible with the right support and self-care. By taking the time to process your emotions, you can find healing and acceptance.

Chapter 6

Recovery and Follow-up

Recovery from myomectomy surgery typically takes around 4 to 6 weeks. During this time, it is important to follow your doctor's instructions for activity restrictions and medications. You may need to take antibiotics to prevent infection and pain medications to help manage any discomfort. Your doctor will likely also recommend that you avoid lifting or straining for several weeks.

To ensure proper healing, you should attend your follow-up appointments. Your doctor will likely check for signs of infection and assess your healing process. They may also discuss any lifestyle changes or medications you may need to make to support healing.

Your doctor may also recommend that you use a heating pad or take warm baths to help manage pain and discomfort. They may also recommend that you take extra care to prevent constipation, which can be a complication of myomectomy surgery.

It is also important to watch for signs of infection, such as fever, redness, swelling, or pain at the incision site. Immediately contact your doctor if you see any of these symptoms.

Finally, if you had a laparoscopic myomectomy, your doctor may recommend that you avoid sexual intercourse until your follow-up appointment. This is to prevent any potential complications.

By following your doctor's instructions and attending all of your follow-up appointments, you can ensure a successful recovery from myomectomy surgery.

Hospital Stay

The length of a hospital stay after a myomectomy surgery will vary depending on the individual's condition and the type of myomectomy procedure that was performed. Typically, a patient can expect to stay in the hospital for 2-3 days after the procedure. Some myomectomy surgeries may require a longer hospital stay, while others may allow the patient to go home on the same day as the procedure. After leaving the hospital, the patient should plan to rest for at least one week before returning to normal activities, and the patient should follow the surgeon's instructions for follow-up care.

It is important for myomectomy patients to take it easy during the recovery period and to follow all the instructions provided by the healthcare team. It is also important to take the necessary precautions to reduce the risk of infection and to ensure that the patient is healing properly.

Follow-up Appointments

Follow-up appointments after a myomectomy surgery are very important. During the appointment, your doctor will want to check your progress since the procedure and make sure that you are healing properly. Your doctor may also want to discuss any possible side effects or complications that may have occurred during or after the surgery. Additionally, your doctor may want to talk to you about any lifestyle changes that may be necessary to help you heal and prevent any future complications.

Diet

1. Increase fiber intake to help keep your digestive system moving and reduce the risk of constipation.

2. Include plenty of fresh fruits and vegetables in your diet, as they are high in nutrients and fiber.

3. Choose lean proteins such as skinless chicken, fish, and tofu to help your body heal.

4. Avoid processed, sugary, and fried foods.

5. Consume calcium-rich foods such as dairy products, fortified cereals and juices, and dark leafy greens to help keep your bones strong.

6. Drink plenty of fluids such as water, herbal teas, and low-fat milk to stay hydrated and help your body heal.

7. Ask your doctor about taking a multivitamin and mineral supplement to ensure you are getting all the necessary nutrients for recovery.

Activity

Your doctor will give you specific instructions on what activities you can do after myomectomy surgery. Generally, you should expect to take about six weeks off from work and limit physical activity during that time. You should avoid heavy lifting and strenuous exercise until your doctor gives you the go-ahead.

You may be able to take short walks around your house or in the neighborhood. It's crucial to pay attention to your body's needs and take it easy If you experience pain or discomfort, rest until it subsides.

When your doctor approves, you can slowly resume your normal activities. Make sure to start with low-impact activities like swimming or walking. As you progress, you can add more strenuous activities like running, biking, or lifting weights.

If you experience any pain or discomfort during activity, stop and rest. You may need to take it slow and adjust the intensity of your activity based on how you feel.

It is important to follow your doctor's instructions and take the time to properly recover after surgery. This will help ensure a successful recovery and reduce your risk of complications.

Chapter 7

Conclusion

Myomectomy surgery is a major surgical procedure, and it is important to discuss the risks and benefits with a medical professional before deciding if it is the right option for you. While it can be a difficult decision, myomectomy surgery can provide relief from a variety of symptoms, and it can help preserve fertility and reduce the risk of complications from fibroids. While there are risks involved, the benefits of this surgery far outweigh the risks for many women. With the help of an experienced medical team and careful consideration of the risks and benefits, myomectomy surgery may be the best choice for you.

Ultimately, myomectomy surgery can be a powerful tool in the fight against fibroids and the symptoms associated with them. It can provide relief from a variety of symptoms, help preserve fertility, and reduce the risk of complications from fibroids. The decision to undergo myomectomy surgery should not be taken lightly, but with careful consideration of the risks and benefits and the help of a qualified medical team, it can be a life-changing procedure for many women.

Made in the USA
Columbia, SC
20 October 2023

24691329R20017